WEIGHT LOSS

30 Tips On How To Lose Weight Fast Without Pills Or Surgery

Weight Loss Motivation And Fat Burning Strategies

BY SANDRA WILLIAMS

Table of Contents

Introduction 4

    [Your Free Gift] 5

Chapter 1: Dietary Tips And Tricks To Lose Weight 8

Chapter 2: Exercise Tips and Tricks to Lose Weight 11

Chapter 3: Lifestyle Tips and Tricks to Lose Weight 14

Chapter 4: Mental Tips and Tricks to Lose Weight 17

Chapter 5: Tips to Ensure that You Remain Motivated 20

Chapter 6: Bonus Tips 23

Conclusion 31

    Would You Like to Know More? 32

[BONUS] 33

    Preview of My Other Book, Wheat Belly Diet 33

    Check Out My Other Books 35

Introduction

I want to thank you and congratulate you for purchasing the book *"Weight Loss - 30 Tips On How To Lose Weight Fast Without Pills Or Surgery, Weight Loss Motivation And Fat Burning Strategies"*.

This book contains all the information you need to lose weight without any surgery or pills.

Are you having a hard time losing weight despite trying numerous diets? Do you find yourself losing weight when on a certain weight loss program only to gain all the weight lost? Do you know that you can actually lose weight without having to starve yourself?

If you are having a hard time losing weight, you have just come to the right place. This book has some ingenious tips that will not make you have to starve or have to hit the gym six days a week just to lose the weight. You only need to incorporate some interesting tips to your diet, exercise program and lifestyle and you will be well on your way to having that dream body you very much desire.

Thanks again for purchasing this book, I hope you will enjoy it!

[Your Free Gift]

As a way of saying thanks for your purchase, I'm offering 2 free reports that are exclusive to my readers:

To check what are The 101 Tips That Burn Belly Fat Daily go to my page here:

=> http://projecteasylife.com/101tips <=

To see what are The 7 (Quick & Easy) Cooking Tricks To Banish Your Boring Diet go to my website here:

=> http://projecteasylife.com/7-tricks <=

© **Copyright 2014 by Sandra Williams - All rights reserved.**

This document is geared towards providing exact and reliable information in regards to the topic and issue covered. The publication is sold with the idea that the publisher is not required to render accounting, officially permitted, or otherwise, qualified services. If advice is necessary, legal or professional, a practiced individual in the profession should be ordered.

From a Declaration of Principles which was accepted and approved equally by a Committee of the American Bar Association and a Committee of Publishers and Associations.

In no way is it legal to reproduce, duplicate, or transmit any part of this document in either electronic means or in printed format. Recording of this publication is strictly prohibited and any storage of this document is not allowed unless with written permission from the publisher. All rights reserved.

The information provided herein is stated to be truthful and consistent, in that any liability, in terms of inattention or otherwise, by any usage or abuse of any policies, processes, or directions contained within is the solitary and utter responsibility of the recipient reader. Under no circumstances will any legal responsibility or blame be held against the publisher for any reparation, damages, or monetary loss due to the information herein, either directly or indirectly.

Respective authors own all copyrights not held by the publisher.

The information herein is offered for informational purposes solely, and is universal as so. The presentation of the information is without contract or any type of guarantee assurance.

The trademarks that are used are without any consent, and the publication of the trademark is without permission or backing by the trademark owner. All trademarks and brands within this book are for clarifying purposes only and are the owned by the owners themselves, not affiliated with this document.

DISCLAIMER: The purpose of this book is to provide information only. The information, though believed to be entirely accurate, is NOT a substitution for medical, psychological or professional advice, diagnosis or treatment. The author recommends that you seek the advice of your physician or other qualified health care provider to present them with questions you may have regarding any medical condition. Advice from your trusted, professional medical advisor should always supersede information presented in this book.

Chapter 1: Dietary Tips And Tricks To Lose Weight

Diet is a very important part of weight loss. We cannot talk about weight loss and fail to mention diet, however much you may not like this. While we all know that you need to eat healthy and nutritious dense foods as well as eat less than your daily calorie intake in order to lose weight, the greatest challenge for many is actually doing this. Therefore, we will look at ingenious ways to eat less so that you can lose weight.

Go Cayenne

Are you aware that you can actually lose weight by eating spicy food? Anytime you put a half teaspoon of cayenne pepper in a bowl of soup, you will in turn eat 60-70 fewer calories in your next meal. Scientists say that cayenne helps boost your metabolism significantly anytime it is consumed in food. However, ensure you have it in the right proportions because too little of it will be negligible and won't have any impact at all.

Drink Olive Oil

In The Shangri-La Diet, author Seth Roberts affirms that you can lose weight by simply taking two tablespoons of olive oil. This is to be done in between meals because this intake of olive oil can actually lower your appetite significantly. This is because consuming flavor-rich foods, which are familiar to you will make your brain stimulate hunger which will see you eat a lot and gain weight. Eating foods with unfamiliar tastes makes your body starve because of brain impulses thereby lowering set points and causing weight loss.

Take Some Vitamin

The International Journal of Obesity conducted a study on 96 obese people with calcium and multi-vitamin supplements. The study went through for twenty-six weeks and the vitamin group ended up with significantly lower body fat than their counterparts. The study concluded that people eat more food because there are certain vitamins or nutrients they are lacking in so their bodies are looking for these nutrients. Therefore, taking adequate vitamins and ensuring that you have no deficit will reduce cravings that may be due to lacking certain nutrients and minerals.

Eat A Heavier Breakfast Than Dinner

In a research done by "The Doctors" with 100 obese women, one group took 200 calories for breakfast and 700 calories for dinner. The other group had 700 calories in the morning, 500 for lunch and an additional 200 for dinner. It was then clear that the group, which took a heavy breakfast shed 20 pounds after a 13 month watch.

How is this possible you may ask? Eating a heavy breakfast gives the body all the energy it needs to start the day. Can you imagine you have not been eating for 6-8 hours when you were sleeping? So, once you wake up, your body is deprived of important nutrients and depriving even more by not taking breakfast will only lead to cravings, you will also be grumpy hence, the need to take comfort food to feel good. You are also likely to binge eat because you will be telling yourself that you did not take breakfast. You will feel justified to eat more.

Drink Red Wine

In 2010, a study in Brigham with 19,000 people showed that ladies who drank at least one glass of wine per day recorded a reduction in weight. They lost relatively more pounds than the non-drinkers did. The same study also indicated that heavy drinkers had a slight weight gain whereas non-drinkers had rapid weight gain. Having a glass of wine after a meal is actually good for you. The best wine is red wine, which is rich in antioxidants.

Drink Plenty Of Water

Do you know that you cannot survive for more than three days without water, while you can survive for longer without taking food and only taking water? This means that water is the core of our survival. So, how does water help you lose weight? Water is essential as sometimes when you think you are hungry and you take a snack, you could actually only be thirsty. Therefore, taking water frequently will eliminate the times when you have to take a snack when you are only thirsty. Additionally, in order for our body to function well in burning fat and getting rid of toxins, it needs water. So, you cannot claim that you want to lose weight when you do not take enough water. Ensure you drink eight glasses of water each day and see the amazing benefits you will enjoy.

Chapter 2: Exercise Tips and Tricks to Lose Weight

The other very important part to losing weight is exercising. You cannot expect to lose weight if you do not exercise. We will look at some exercise tips that will help you lose weight.

Skip Through Commercials

Always get moving. As you watch your favorite TV show, and there is a commercial break, you can always dance, skip, go up or down the stairs continuously. All you need to do is to find something that will get your heartbeat up such that you feel somewhat breathless. If you do this with just a 2 minute break for a TV night of 2 hours you will burn an extra 270 calories. This will translate to 28 pounds for the year in lost weight. It may seem small but it is better than nothing.

Add Mini-Strength Training

Most weight loss exercises such as push-ups or squats are simply ways of building up one's metabolism to the calorie burning levels. They are just as effective as hitting the gym. The basic rule of exercising is to fatigue your muscles within first 90 seconds. Consider 10 reps of squats, lunges, chair dips, crunches and knee push-ups. Gradually increase the reps that it takes for your muscles to be fatigued.

Walk 5 Minutes More

An increased daily activity by just a few minutes significantly reflects on your overall weight loss. If your goal is to do an hour of exercise, say walking or jogging per session, then you can always increase this by just five minutes and you will realize the change. You will burn off an extra 120 calories every day, which will amount to 13 pounds a year.

Climb Extra Stairs

If you have a choice between climbing and riding, then climbing is the best for weight loss. Cover about five floors each day with 3 minute stair climbing. Doing this continuously will eliminate the average weight gain per year of one pound. Generally climbing stairs is also good for your health and it's an effective exercise to shed some pounds in your butt or waistline. Studies have it that men who climb over 70 stairs each week have a reduction in mortality rate by 20%. You can always start with just a few stairs every day and increase on the numbers over time.

Jog For Junk Mail

You can turn your clutter into a challenge easily. Make it a habit that for each mail you pull from your mailbox every day, you do a lap round your building. Alternatively, you can always go up and down the stairs. Each session will see you burn up to 140 calories.

Make The Most Out Of Your Walk

Many people have a routine of walking, which is commendable. If you like walking, ensure you make the best out of the walking sessions. Increase your effort by finding challenges like walking on a hill. Just ensure the challenges come in at the beginning of your walk because that's when you will have a lot of energy to spare and challenge yourself. You can also engage your kids during the walk, as they will get playful and make you chase them. Your dog is also a perfect option so long as he or she can run fast as you chase him or her.

Chapter 3: Lifestyle Tips and Tricks to Lose Weight

Sleep Away The Weight Gain

Sleep earlier than usual and you will realize weight loss in just a week. Poor sleeping habits causes weight gain according to a study conducted by the University of Pennsylvania. People who are deprived of sleep gain almost 3 pounds compared to well-rested people who actually lose weight. This is because when you do not sleep better, you tend to be grumpy, make poor food choices because of the need to find comfort from the food as well as lack adequate energy to exercise. So, now you can see how your sleeping late is affecting your ability to lose weight.

Watch Less TV

On average, adults watch TV for five hours each day. Watching TV not only makes you inactive but also exposes you to the many food commercials. Such commercials make you desire certain foods that the TV may bring out as cool. Additionally, if you watch TV and see the glamorous lives celebrities live, you become depressed. This might in turn make you to turn to food to seek some comfort, which only leads to weight gain.

Eat Using Smaller Plates

Avoid big bowls and large plates, which can accommodate too much food. Instead, use smaller plates. The good thing is that even if you fill up a smaller plate, the quantity of food is much less as compared to if you filled a large plate with food. Furthermore, if you are trying to lose weight, you are unlikely to fill the plate with food because you think that it is too much. Over time, your stomach will get used to the smaller quantities and this will translate to greater weight loss.

Make Your Own Meals

A sample premade chicken from chain restaurants contains 600 calories and almost 50% of the calories come from fat. The chicken also has more than half of the daily requirement of sodium, 1440mg. You can always make your own chicken sandwich with some whole wheat bread, some lettuce and light mayo for just 230 calories. In total, you will cut over 500mg of sodium and an additional 400 calories. With the self-prepared meal, you will have some space for salad, that can add up to 28 pounds of weight loss in a year. Making your own food does not only put you in control of what you eat but also makes you reduce the amount of salt, fat and sugar that you take in. Restaurants have a higher count of some unwanted nutrients.

Doggie Bag The Dinner

If you really have to eat at a restaurant or a fast food joint, ask the waiter to divide your food into two and pack the other half. Restaurants are usually very notorious for serving large amounts of food. This way, you will not feel compelled to eat all the food you are served in one sitting.

Don't Multi Task As You Eat

Engaging in some other activity as you eat will distract you. If you are fond of watching TV, working or reading as you eat then you are likely to not pay much attention to what you take in. Moreover, you will not be enjoying each bite because your mind will be distracted. Take your time, serve your food and sit down to eat it. Pay close attention to the textures and flavors by chewing slowly. This way, you will really enjoy your food and not end up eating mindlessly.

Bring Lunch To Work Tomorrow

Ensure you have packed lunch. When you pack your lunch, you practice portion control and know your sizes. It is better than having your lunch at the cafe or a fast food joint next to the office. Takeaways contain many calories even though they are convenient. Besides, they are also very expensive compared to packed lunch.

Chapter 4: Mental Tips and Tricks to Lose Weight

In addition to exercising, eating well, and making some lifestyle changes, you also need some mental tips and tricks to lose weight.

Never Eat In Your Pajamas

Wearing baggy clothing will always make you want more food. Avoid your baggy lounge pants or pajamas when eating. Loose clothing gives you a bad perception and illusions of staying slimmer and averts your thinking from calories. Wearing fitted clothes makes you more concerned and cautious about your figure even though it's not advisable to wear restrictive clothes. When wearing fitting clothes, you will certainly know when you should stop eating some foods and be in control of your weight.

Ditch All Or Nothing Thinking

With all or nothing thinking, you are likely to make unreasonable goals which will be difficult to achieve. Even a 20 pound loss instead of 100 is still significant. Don't be too obsessed about hitting an insanely huge target; instead, you should learn to enjoy the journey and not the destination. Focus on the little you achieve and build on it day by day.

Sniff Vanilla

Are sugar cravings ruining your dieting resolve? If yes, then the best suggestion is to light a spritze or vanilla candle which is scented. Alternatively, you can put the vanilla scented patch on the back of your hand. The smell of vanilla will certainly help you stay slim because it reduces your cravings and appetite for sugar and other sweet things.

Take A Picture Of Your Food Before Eating

Have the habit of always taking a photo of your food before you can eat. Once you finish eating, you can look at the picture and see how much you have actually eaten. Once you see how much you have eaten, you will be embarrassed and the next time you would not want to eat as much.

Surround Yourself With Blue

Did you know that the color blue is an appetite suppressant? This is the reason why most restaurants and fast food joints are not painted in blue. If you were placed in a blue room with your best food, you will have 33% less. Apparently, the blue light makes your food look less appealing. Therefore, as you eat, ensure you are dressed in blue, eat in blue plates and have a table cloth that is blue in color. Colors that encourage eating and increase one's appetite are orange, yellow and red. You are advised to avoid them.

Eat With Less Favored Hand

A study was conducted on 1000 teens who frequent movies. It was observed that those who were at the movies and ate popcorns with their less favored hand ended up consuming less. The Journal of Personality & Social Psychology also confirmed the findings to be very true. Generally, eating with your non-dominant hand makes you consume less. Even though it doesn't feel natural, you are not likely to eat mindlessly. If you want to lose weight, you can try this out immediately.

Chapter 5: Tips to Ensure that You Remain Motivated

Motivation is crucial to any person who wants to lose weight. You need that motivation to go the extra mile even when you don't feel like exercising or you just want to eat that whole bowl of ice cream. Let us look at some tips to get you motivated in your weight loss journey.

Showcase Your Photos

Take a photo of yourself and display it somewhere you can see it all the time. This way, you can know and be aware of the fact that you are getting bigger. This should give you enough motivation to do something to shed those unwanted pounds. After you have made some progress, take another photo of yourself then post it next to the one you had. Repeat this process until you get to your desired weight. Just knowing how far you have come will serve as enough motivation to help you get going.

Revisit The Disadvantages Of Being Overweight

When you are overweight or obese, you must get comments from people about your weight. Such comments are always embarrassing and hard to get over. It is advisable to keep those comments that you got during the moments when you overweight ringing in your mind so that you can keep going and work even harder. Revisit situations when friends, siblings or children were embarrassed of your weight and take it upon yourself to make them proud by shedding off some pounds.

Seize Your Strength

Take your time and stand naked in front of a mirror after every few days. Identify your favorite body part and analyze how that part has been affected by your weight. Work towards ensuring that the specific body part comes back to normal and you will realize you like it more. If it's your butt, then you will love it as you lose more pounds. Also, convince yourself that you are not meant to be overweight forever and you will get the motivation to go on.

Celebrate Each Victory

After observing all the precautions and the recommendations until you realize some result, it's advisable to celebrate. Don't be so rigid. Losing all those 50 pounds is an achievement. Reward yourself with a trip to the movies or buy your favorite dress. Always remember that each pound lost is worth celebrating always.

Set Small Goals

Take your notebook and a pen. Write down the small goals you would really love to achieve. The mini goals are very important to keep you going. Ensure the goals range from your eating habits to your overall lifestyle. Some of your goals can be:

- Giving up on alcohol completely or having it during the weekends only.
- Having more veggies and fruits on a daily basis.
- Walking up the stairs all the time without gasping. Also, give up on elevators and escalators.
- Going for side salads instead of fries.
- Frequenting exercises for at least thirty minutes each day.

Start small and grow with the changes. It is practically very difficult to initiate all the changes you can imagine of because your brain will definitely not want the change since as human beings, we are resistant to change. Therefore, make small changes and gradually improve your life.

Take Your Measurements

For now, your statistics might not be very appealing to you. However, in future you will be very pleased to write down the number of pounds you have lost in just a few weeks. Taking the measurements and seeing how many inches you have lost is a perfect way of measuring your success. Also, note that measuring is very different from looking at the scale because sometimes the scale won't go down but the measurements on your body will.

Chapter 6: Bonus Tips

Herb It Up

Stock up some herbs in your spice rack. Alternatively, you can have a small herb garden in your kitchen window. Herbs, just like spices, are amazing flavor additives that can keep your appetite in check.

Tone Your Tummy While You Sit

When sitting, you can make small moves that will make a difference in your weight. The American Dietetic Association observed that contracting and relaxing your muscles when you watch TV or when you drive for at least half an hour actually works. You will certainly feel some slight pain the next day but it's actually worth it.

Add Resistance

Resistance training functions better than doing cardio alone. If you lift free weights and follow that up with cardio, you will lose more pounds. However, you have to lift the free weight first because your muscles need some boost for them to perform well. Depleting all the energy you had in aerobics alone will not give you enough weight benefits from weight training.

Sweat It Out

Exercise is efficient in losing weight. Calorie intake also plays a similar role. However, sweating it out ensures that your mental and cardiovascular health is well taken care of. Mixing cardio and toning at least five times a week will always keep your metabolism on the high for some time.

Eat After Exercise

Taking proteins just after exercise sessions helps you burn more fat. In fact, you will not lose your lean muscle. Having a recovery shake ensures that you will improve in your next training session and that you will not have unnecessary injuries. In one cup of milk, add 13g of protein powder then add in some three ice cubes. You can also substitute this with any other protein smoothie, as it will be digested quickly and deliver the required nutrients faster for the purposes of building muscles.

Avoid Carbs Before Workout Sessions

If your focus is exercise-induced weight loss then you have to ensure you don't eat carbs at least 2 hours before the workout session. A study by Dan Goldberg, personal trainer at Health Fitness Forum, showed that bikers who skipped carbs for the 2 hours 30 minutes before the ride lost more fats. Those who had carb-rich snacks did not burn as much fat. You can have low fat yogurt or chocolate milk.

Obey The 1-Mile Rule

Each additional hour you spend in your car driving increases your obesity by 6%. The one mile rule ensures that you burn calories instead of gas. If you have errands that are just a mile away, you can always walk all the way. Alternatively, you can also park where you will be able to run different errands within a one mile radius. If you walk each day, you will be 17 pounds lighter next year.

Cover The Clock When Exercising

When you exercise and keep staring at the clock, you lose the motivation and zeal to keep going. Assuming there were no clocks to watch is a handy strategy for ensuring that you exercise more. Therefore, when working out, ensure you cover the clock just so you don't get too cautious of the time. You will realize the time you set had passed a long time ago even though you keep going. It's simple; use your towel or t-shirt to cover the clock.

Sign Up To Facebook

How does Facebook help in weight loss? As weird as it is, simply staring at your screen and staying online on Facebook makes you forget about your hunger. Such a distraction removes food oriented thinking from your mind and in turn helps you lose weight because of low calorie intake.

Sign Up For Newsletters

Both nutritionists and other weight loss experts believe in this technique to be very efficient. People who receive weekly or fortnight newsletters about weight and fitness will certainly increase their activity over time. The newsletters can be in form of magazines or emails. Signing up for the newsletters keeps you motivated and makes you focused on shedding pounds especially when your morale is fading quickly. Some of the newsletters are "Eat Up, Slim Down", "Exercise of the Week" and "400 Calorie Fix".

Get A Dose Of Laughter

Laughter is perfect for not only mood boost but also keeps your blood sugar in check. Researchers at the University of Tsukuba in Japan discovered that people who watched funny clips and were happier had a low blood sugar level compared to those who didn't. Giggling, for example, works your tummy muscles and in turn processes glucose faster. A stable sugar level in your blood controls your appetite. You might need to put your funniest pal on speed dial for you to lose some pounds.

Make Use Of Chopsticks

The main advantage of chopsticks is that they make you mindful of whatever goes through your mouth. Many people don't know how to use chopsticks and if you are one of them then you are better off learning because using them will force you to be mindful. It is too hard to pile up foods between two wooden sticks.

Sleep In A Cold Room

Chills make the body adjust to speedy metabolism. Your sleep will also be improved significantly. When you sleep in a cold room, you unknowingly make your body to heat up and keep yourself warm for numerous hours. As your body heats up, it burns down calories fast.

Tie One On

It is a French fashion culture to tie a ribbon under the waist when the ladies go out for dinner. You can emulate this and succeed in your weight loss initiative. The ribbon keeps you conscious of your tummy. As the evening goes on, you will realize that the ribbon gets tighter and tighter. You will therefore know when to stop eating and feasting.

Use A Symbol

The best symbol you can use is that nice dress, pants or t-shirt that you can no longer fit into. Hang it somewhere you can see it all the time and take it upon yourself to fit into the dress after you achieve your goal weight. A symbol is beneficial as it always reminds you of your goal and gives you the motivation to keep on going despite the challenges.

Eat At The End Of The Table

When you are at a party, develop the habit of eating at the end of a table. While you are at the end, your favorite dishes become less accessible and you are not likely to shout for food in public.

Eat In Front Of A Mirror

As you eat, stay relaxed and have a mirror in front of you. As you watch yourself eat, you become very cautious and conscious of what you take in. Thus, you will end up taking little amounts of food, which in turn means that you will control your eating.

Clean Your Closet

This great exercise doubles up as a perfect change of your attitude. You certainly have those clothes that you feel bad about so get rid of them. Throw away anything, which looks big because you are not giving yourself options of ever fitting in the big clothes again. Ensure all the small clothes are at the front because they will act as a motivation to you. Seeing these clothes every day when picking clothes to wear will remind you of your goal.

Grab A Magazine

Anytime you feel the urge to grab something from the fridge, grab a magazine instead. Do this continuously and you will realize that you actually take some time before you get hungry again. Experts say that if you grab a magazine and distract yourself for 15 minutes, a continuous practice will make you distracted for almost 2hours. Your cravings will be delayed even longer as time goes by.

Postpone Any Indulgence

When you see your favorite food, you are likely to cave in and indulge quickly. Fries, steak, or chicken are some of the favorites, which will lead to weight gain. Any time you see them at a cafeteria or any other place, ensure you postpone the indulgence. For example, you can always tell yourself that there is a next time. After some time, you will start asking yourself whether you really need the foods at all. Postponement is very efficient and has been used by many people to keep away from foods that might cause relapse when you are at the peak of your weight loss program.

Leave Something On Your Plate

When having any meal at any given time, practice the habit of leaving some food on your plate. If you make it a habit, you will still feel satisfied by eating a bit less. For example, you can simply have half the sandwich and just several bites of the bagel and not necessarily the whole bagel.

Try The Toothpaste Diet

When you brush your teeth with mint flavored toothpaste every day, your brain adjusts and prefers a clean feel. Minty fresh tastes have been known to help you stick to the weight loss diet. Brush your teeth at least twice each day so that you can control your snacking. Moreover, brushing teeth helps maintain clean teeth and prevent tooth decay or toothache.

Make A Dream Book

A dream book is supposed to have your pictures before you gained all that weight. It's also supposed to have pictures of friends, celebrities or any other person you admire and want to look like. The dream book will build your confidence and make you work harder as you try losing weight. Looking and admiring people who have lost weight could actually make you work harder to be like such people.

Schedule Nudges

Have a calendar full of upcoming events and important occasions. Be aware of all the friends or family who will come into town in the next few days. When you think about having pizza or junk, your mind will go straight to the events. Soon, how you will look at the event will matter more than the food. Anytime you almost slide into binge eating, think of the events and how too much food would ruin your good looks.

Conclusion

Thank you again for purchasing this book!

Losing weight is one of the hardest things for many people. However, this does not mean that losing weight is not possible. With the right kind of motivation and having a plan as to how you are going to eat and exercise, then you are set to shed those extra pounds.

I hope this book has helped you know some ingenious tips that will certainly help you lose weight.

Now I would like to ask for a *small* favor. I am self-published author, and if you liked my book, a review on Amazon would be a great help for me. This feedback will let me continue to write the kind of books that will help people and will let me improve.

Go to http://bit.ly/weightlosstipsreview to review, and thanks in advance for any kind of support!

Thank you and good luck!

– Sandra

Would You Like to Know More?

To check what are The 101 Tips That Burn Belly Fat Daily go to my page here:

=> http://projecteasylife.com/101tips <=

To see what are The 7 (Quick & Easy) Cooking Tricks To Banish Your Boring Diet go to my website here:

=> http://projecteasylife.com/7-tricks <=

[BONUS]

Preview of My Other Book, Wheat Belly Diet
(…)

Why Use the Wheat Belly Diet for the Best Results?

If you have tried and failed with other diets, perhaps you were not eliminating the right types of foods. Rethinking wheat has helped people to eliminate the harm it causes to your body. Getting rid of belly fat has thus far been a successful goal for people using the Wheat-Belly Diet.

Very few wheat-based foods are actually healthy for you to eat. The wheat used today, which Dr. Davis calls "Frankenwheat", is genetically modified, and it isn't the same wheat that your parents used to eat.

The modification of the wheat plant has allowed it to be thicker and shorter, so that it is more beneficial for farmers, and more resistant to disease. The bad aspect of this wheat is that it is not as nutritionally rich as conventional wheat, and can damage your health.

The glycemic index is higher in today's wheat than it is in sugar. Some candy bars have a healthier glycemic index than a slice of wheat bread. Glutens that are present in larger amounts in today's wheat cause cravings, and that leads to excess belly fat.

Dr. Davis says that you can expect better results from a wheat-free meal plan, because wheat is more than simply a gluten source. "Frankenwheat" affects the mind, by stimulating your appetite and it can cause depression and anxiety, especially for people who are overweight.

Giving up wheat will allow you to lose belly fat, and can also help in other health issues, such as those mentioned above. People are finally beginning to see the negative effects of today's wheat on their health, and those who stay with the Wheat Belly Diet often find benefits that they did not even expect.

(…)

To check out the rest of the book ***Wheat Belly Diet***, go to Amazon here: http://bit.ly/wheatbellydiet

Check Out My Other Books

Below you'll find some of my other books that are popular on Amazon and Kindle as well. Simply go to the links below to check them out. Alternatively, you can visit my author page on Amazon to see other work done by me:

Author page: http://bit.ly/SandraWilliams

Gluten Free And Wheat Free Total Health Revolution

Wheat Belly Cookbook – 37 Wheat Free Recipes To Lose The Wheat And Have All-Day Energy (http://bit.ly/bellycookbook)

Gluten Free – The Gluten Free Diet For Beginners Guide, What Is Celiac Disease, How To Eat Healthier And Have More Energy (http://bit.ly/glutenfreebook)

Gluten Free Cookbook – 30 Healthy And Easy Gluten Free Recipes For Beginners, Gluten Free Diet Plan For A Healthy Lifestyle (http://bit.ly/gfreecookbook)

How To REALLY Set And Achieve Goals

Goals – Setting And Achieving S.M.A.R.T. Goals, How To Stay Motivated And Get Everything You Want From Your Life Faster (http://bit.ly/getsmartgoals)

Prevent And Reverse Diabetes Disease

Diabetes – Diabetes Prevention And Symptoms Reversing (http://bit.ly/diabetesguide)

Diabetic Cookbook – 30 Diabetes Diet Recipes For Diabetic Living, Control Low Sugar And Reverse Diabetes Naturally (http://bit.ly/diabetic-cookbook)

Get Healthy, Have More Energy And Live Longer With Natural Paleo And Mediterranean Foods

Paleo – *The Paleo Diet For Beginners Guide, Easy And Practical Solution For Weight Loss And Healthy Eating* (http://bit.ly/healthypaleo)

Paleo Cookbook – *30 Healthy And Easy Paleo Diet Recipes For Beginners, Start Eating Healthy And Get More Energy With Practical Paleo Approach* (http://bit.ly/tastypaleo)

Mediterranean Diet – *Easy Guide To Healthy Life With Mediterranean Cuisine, Fast And Natural Weight Loss For Beginners* (http://bit.ly/mediterraneanbook)

Mediterranean Diet Cookbook – *30 Healthy And Easy Mediterranean Diet Recipes For Beginners* (http://bit.ly/mediterracookbook)

Extremely Fast Weight Loss With Low Carb Approach

Ketogenic Diet – *Easy Keto Diet Guide For Healthy Life And Fast Weight Loss, Heal Yourself And Get More Energy With Low Carb Diet* (http://bit.ly/ketodietbook)

Ketogenic Diet Cookbook – *30 Keto Diet Recipes For Beginners, Easy Low Carb Plan For A Healthy Lifestyle And Quick Weight Loss* (http://bit.ly/ketocookbook)

Atkins Cookbook – *30 Quick And Easy Atkins Diet Recipes For Beginners, Plan Your Low Carb Days With The New Atkins Diet Book* (http://bit.ly/atkinscookbook)

Amazing Weight Loss Tips, Tricks And Motivation

Ultimate Guide To Diets – *Choose The Best Diet For Your Body, Live Healthy And Happy Life Without Supplements And Pills* (http://bit.ly/dietsbook)

The Obesity Cure *– How To Lose Weight Fast And Overcome Obesity Forever* (http://bit.ly/obesitybook)

Unique Beauty Tips Every Woman Should Know

Younger Next Month *– Anti-Aging Guide For Women* (http://bit.ly/beyoungerbook)

Hair Care And Hair Growth Solutions *– How To Regrow Your Hair Faster, Hair Loss Treatment And Hair Growth Remedies* (http://bit.ly/haircarebook)

Improve State Of Mind, Defeat Bad Feelings And Be Happy!

Anxiety Workbook *– Free Cure For Anxiety Disorder And Depression Symptoms, Panic Attacks And Social Anxiety Relief Without Medication And Pills* (http://bit.ly/anxietybook)

The Depression Cure *– Depression Self Help Workbook, Cure And Free Yourself From Depression Naturally And For Life* (http://bit.ly/depressioncurebook)

If the links do not work, for whatever reason, you can simply search for the titles on the Amazon website to find them. Best regards!

Manufactured by Amazon.ca
Bolton, ON